50 NATURAL WAYS TO
RELIEVE PMS

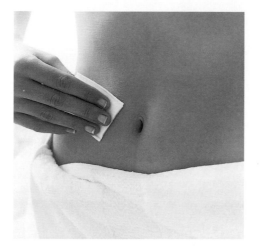

50 NATURAL WAYS TO
RELIEVE PMS

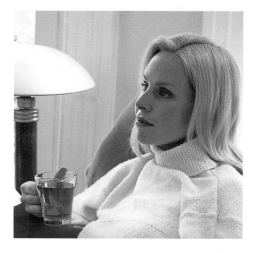

Practical quick-fix tips to help prevent and
alleviate the physical and mental
symptoms of PMS

Tracey Kelly

LORENZ BOOKS

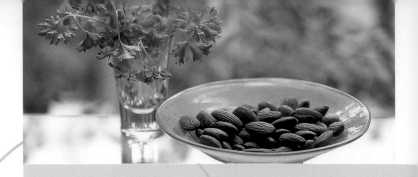

contents

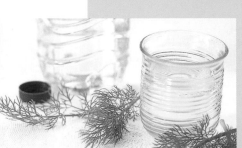

50 NATURAL WAYS TO
RELIEVE PMS

Spending time with people who give you confidence and support is important at this time of the month.

introduction

Many women dread two weeks out of every month, from the time of ovulation right through to the start of menstruation. Most experience, to some degree, at least some of the large number of symptoms that make up premenstrual syndrome (PMS), from mild discomfort and food cravings, to painful abdominal cramps, headaches and migraine, water retention, nasal congestion or aching limbs.

nutritional aids
Fortunately, there are many ways to alleviate, if not eradicate, PMS conditions. Taking steps to control your diet alone can yield vast improvements. Making sure that you eat a small portion of starchy food every few hours, and taking care to avoid caffeine, alcohol, high-fat and high-sugar foods, will keep your blood sugar on an even keel. This will act to control mood swings and

prevent migraines, for example. Fruit juices and smoothies will help curb a tendency to binge on sweet foods, while yogurt containing "friendly" bacteria will help balance the bacteria in your stomach, making for fewer episodes of indigestion and bloating.

Including all the essential vitamins and minerals in your diet – from cramp-relieving vitamin B6 to magnesium, which reduces sugar and chocolate cravings – will go a long way to keeping you feeling your best.

Over the long term, taking supplements such as evening primrose oil and borage oil, which contain essential fatty acids (EFAs), can help balance your hormonal levels and control a wide range of symptoms. Herbal supplements such as feverfew for headaches and peppermint for stomach upsets provide immediate relief.

healthful exercise

Exercise is, of course, important at any time of the month, but it is crucial to stretch the muscles when you are experiencing PMS achiness and tenderness in the tissues. You can reduce high-impact exercises at times when you are feeling tender, and concentrate on gentle stretches, such as Pilates and yoga. Add some simple exercises designed specifically to alleviate discomfort in areas such as the abdomen and back. The legs are another area where it is common to experience premenstrual discomfort; stretching the muscles will ease pain, especially when you are sitting at a desk or at bedtime.

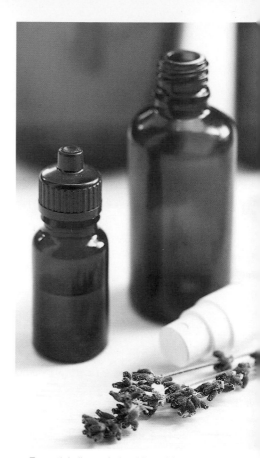

▲ Essential oils can help with a wide range of symptoms, both physical and mental.

soothing treatments

Treatments that use aromatherapy can go a long way towards relieving symptoms. Essential oils such as pine, crampbark and rosemary can soothe painful tissues, while oils such as clary sage and naiouli have been known to help balance female hormones. Incense mixtures can help you achieve a state of calm when your nerves are frayed and you are feeling irritable, and gentle inhalations can ease the sinus congestion and asthma that many women experience during the days preceding menstruation. A dose of pure pleasure, flower oils such as rose and jasmine can help raise the spirits with their delicious and enlivening scents.

palliative measures

There are many therapies that will not only soothe physical discomfort, but also act as system "rechargers". Reflexology is good for relieving built-up pressure in the ovaries, and an abdomen massage will ease cramps, working from the outside in. By practising deep breathing, you will be oxygenating all the cells in your body, thus improving the function of its systems. Solutions such

as homeopathy and crystal healing can balance both physical and emotional systems, while Reiki works by directing a positive flow of fast-acting, healing energy from one person to another – and you can also train to use it on yourself.

uplifting attitudes

By keeping a simple chart of your symptoms each month, you can get some idea of the impact PMS has on your life. This will help remind you of why you may not feel your best, and encourage you to be easy on yourself. It will also help you plan important activities for the more high-energy days of the month.

Daily positive affirmations can help boost your confidence levels, while taking measures to enjoy sex fully at a time when your libido level is high can enhance your relationship with your partner. In the modern world, we tend to forget our physical links with nature, but understanding the effect the lunar cycle has on women can be a real eye-opener.

If you get over-emotional, then meditation can help you maintain calm and perspective, as can sound, peaceful sleep at night. The more vivid dreams that accompany this time of heightened awareness can help broaden your experience of self, helping you to accept and enjoy this time as an important aspect of life.

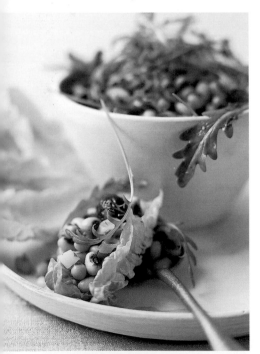

◄ *Legumes such as beans provide the slow-burning carbohydrates and high fibre that help to keep your body's blood sugar levels on an even keel.*

▾ Meditation can help you sustain a centred and calm attitude through times when your emotions seem "out of control".

symptom-easing strategies

It is possible to reduce the intensity of premenstrual symptoms by changing the way you eat and drink in the week or so before your period. This book gives you strategies for eating little and often, curbing cravings for sugar and fat, and including nutrients in your diet to ease the discomfort of headaches and migraine, water retention, bloating and tenderness.

Also included are ideas for sensible exercise – from calming yoga to gentle stretches – together with natural therapies that will dispel aches and discomfort in areas such as the back and abdomen. Aromatherapy and herbal treatments not only do wonders for physical symptoms, their fresh scents give you an emotional lift as well.

Because this can be a sensitive time of the month, strategies for dealing with mood swings and handling relationships ensure that minor irritations are dealt with before they become major problems. Finally, tips on boosting your self-esteem and exploring creative activities can help you use this time to your best advantage.

▼ *Make a list of positive affirmations to boost low self-confidence during what may be a sensitive time of the month.*

1

frequent starch diet

Specialists have discovered that following a diet that includes eating starchy food every few hours is the most important thing you can do to keep premenstrual symptoms at bay.

healthy balance

The single most effective and natural way you can help to prevent PMS symptoms is by eating a small amount of starchy food every 3 hours. This will ensure a healthy blood sugar balance, which will in turn ensure that progesterone – an important hormone released by the ovaries and adrenals – is absorbed into the cells. Correct progesterone absorption cannot take place in the cells if adrenaline – the "fight or flight" hormone – is present. If you miss a meal and your blood sugar level dips,

the body suffers from an excess of adrenaline, leading not only to physical symptoms such as water retention and breast tenderness, but also to feelings of irritability, anxiety and confusion.

the diet

Continue to eat well-balanced and nutritious foods, and follow these guidelines during the week before and during a period. Starches to eat include oats, breads, rice, corn, potatoes and rye. They should preferably be whole foods without additives. When you are going out, take snacks with you: if your blood sugar level dips, it takes the body several days to "reclaim" the benefits.
• Morning: eat a starchy food within an hour of waking.
• Daytime: eat a small, starchy snack every 3 hours.
• Evening: eat a starchy food not more than an hour before going to sleep.
• Do not go for more than 10 hours overnight without eating.

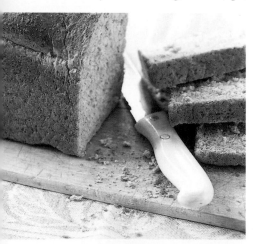

◂ *Keep a fresh loaf of bread on hand so that you can quickly prepare starchy snacks.*

2 binge-curbing foods

It is counterproductive to go on an eating spree at any time, but especially just before your period, when blood sugar levels are best kept on an even keel. Some foods can help to prevent bingeing.

Research has shown that you can help to alleviate premenstrual symptoms by decreasing your intake of refined sugar, chocolate, salt and saturated fats. This may be a time when you find that you crave these types of food the most, but you can curb your appetite for them by having healthier foods on hand and eating regularly throughout the day.

snack bowl

Keep a large bowl handy filled with a selection of fresh fruits – for example, bananas, grapes, apples and pears. Their fructose (fruit sugar) content will curb your appetite for the refined sugars in cakes and cookies. Nuts and seeds are also good to keep at hand: they are extremely nutritious and provide healthy plant oils rather than harmful saturated fats.

All vegetables are storehouses of vitamins and minerals. Chop up some crudités – carrots, celery, green and red peppers, spring onions – and put them in a bowl of iced water so that

they stay fresh and appetizing. Their crunchy texture will satisfy the need to chew, and keep you from grabbing salty, high-fat snacks.

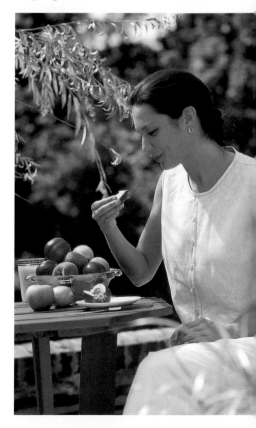

▸ *Fresh fruit is nutritious and will curb your desire for refined sugars.*

3

digestion-aiding yogurt

Stomach upsets can plague PMS sufferers. A simple way to ensure smooth digestion is to include live yogurt in your diet, especially in the week before and during your period.

beneficial bacteria

Live yogurt contains bacteria that aid the essential maintenance of digestive function in the stomach and intestines. These include *Lactobacillus acidophilus* and *Bifidobacteria* cultures.

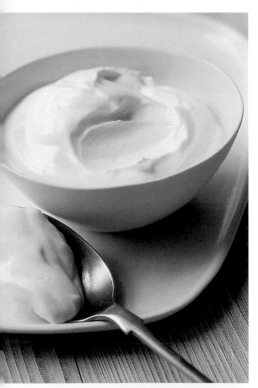

They help the body maintain high levels of "friendly" bacteria and work to prevent intestinal upsets such as yeast infections (sometimes brought on by eating too many sugary foods).

versatile ingredient

If you are not in the habit of eating plain yogurt, you'll be surprised at the number of different ways you can incorporate it into your diet. Apart from the traditional muesli and yogurt for breakfast, you can add fresh fruit and nuts to plain yogurt, blend it with fruit to make thick smoothies, and mix it with fruit juices to make health-giving drinks.

Yogurt also makes a delicious addition to many savoury dishes. Try adding it as a garnish to soups, or mix it with chives for a low-fat topping on baked potatoes. You can add a dash of mustard to yogurt and use it as a dip for crudités or corn chips. Yogurt makes the perfect base for creamy salad dressings to use on green or potato salads.

◂ *You can add fruit to plain yogurt or use it in a variety of savoury dips and dressings.*

4 juices for sugar cravings

Indulging in sugary snacks can send blood sugar levels into orbit during PMS. These healthy juices contain minerals and fructose, burned slowly by the body, to help reduce cravings.

apple and leaf lift-off

This fragrant blend of apple, grapes, fresh leaves and lime juice is a refreshing rejuvenator.

1 apple
150g/5oz white grapes
small handful of fresh coriander (cilantro), with stalks
25g/1oz watercress or rocket (arugula)
15ml/1 tbsp lime juice

Cut the apple into quarters. Using an extractor, juice the apple, grapes, coriander and watercress. Add the lime juice to the fruit and herb mixture and stir. Pour into a glass and drink immediately.

fennel fusion

This aromatic combination is full of minerals and vitamins.

½ small red cabbage
½ fennel bulb
2 apples
15ml/1 tbsp lemon juice

▶ *These juices help to reduce cravings and are a healthy alternative to sweet snacks.*

Slice the red cabbage and the fennel into chunks and cut the apple into quarters. Using an extractor, juice the vegetables and fruit. Stir the lemon juice into the mixture and drink immediately.

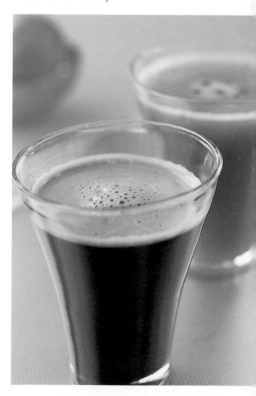

5 cystitis easers

Before and during your period, your urinary tract can be prone to infection. Including cranberry and blueberry in your diet can help prevent cystitis, a bacterial infection of the bladder and urethra.

Cystitis is marked by a burning sensation when urinating, as well as the frequent urge to urinate. It is caused when *E. coli* bacteria bind themselves to the urinary tract lining, and there is an increased tendency for this to occur after sex and during premenstrual and menstruation days. Studies have shown that cranberries can actually inhibit this process, and doctors have long recommended that women include cranberry juice in their diet, both to alleviate and to prevent the condition.

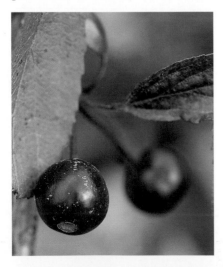

cranberry-blueberry crush
Refreshing cranberries are tart, so you would not want to eat them "straight". Ready-made juices are the easiest option, and are sometimes mixed with apple and raspberry juice. A traditional way to eat the fruit is in cranberry sauce, which is served with turkey, chicken or vegetarian nut roasts.

Blueberries are a powerful antioxidant, and also help to reduce the risk of infection. Milder-tasting than cranberries, they can be added straight to yogurt, muesli and cereals. Whir a handful of blueberries in a blender with cranberry juice and ice for a super, bacteria-busting drink.

supplement options
Because cranberries contain very little sugar, a substantial amount is added to commercial juices. Low-sugar varieties are now available, and cranberry supplements, available from health food stores, are a good way to avoid the extra sugar completely.

◂ *Cranberry juice helps to prevent and ease painful cystitis. It is best to buy ready-made juices because fresh cranberries are tart.*

helpful herbal teas

Some herbs act to ease and dispel a variety of PMS symptoms. Instead of coffee or tea – which contain caffeine, known to increase anxiety and discomfort – try these soothing combinations.

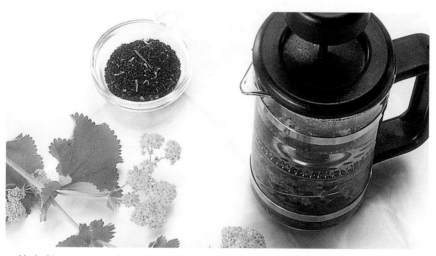

▲ *Herbal teas are a gentle way to relieve PMS symptoms, relax the system and lift the mood.*

lady's mantle and vervain tea

This herbal infusion is said to be effective in the prevention of heavy bleeding during periods.

Put 5ml/1 tsp each of dried lady's mantle and vervain in a pot, then add 300ml/½ pint/1¼ cups boiling water. Steep for 10 minutes, strain and sweeten to taste with honey or brown sugar. Drink one cup twice a day from day 14 of your monthly cycle (two weeks after the beginning of your period).

rose petal and valerian tea

Good for easing premenstrual insomnia, valerian is a potent relaxer. Rose petals ease pain, lift the spirits and smell lovely.

Place 5ml/1 tsp rose petals in a pot with 2.5ml/½ tsp valerian (you can use the powdered contents of a capsule). Add 300ml/½ pint/1¼ cups boiling water and steep for 5–10 minutes. Add a small amount of honey, or drink unsweetened.

Pluck a
sprig of chamomile
fresh from the garden,
add a slice of lemon, pour on
hot water and drink to
calm the nerves and
quell PMS anger.

nutritious vegetables

8

Including plenty of fresh vegetables in your diet will help keep PMS at bay. This dish contains spinach, for calcium and iron (a mineral that is often depleted monthly), and dill to aid digestion.

spinach with rice and dill
Serves 4
675g/1½lb fresh spinach
60ml/4 tbsp extra virgin olive oil
1 large onion, chopped
juice of ½ lemon

150ml/¼ pint/⅔ cup water
115g/4oz long grain rice
45ml/3 tbsp chopped fresh dill, plus
    extra sprigs to garnish
ground black pepper
salt

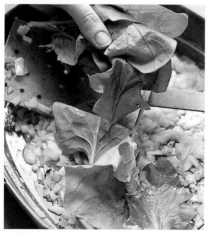

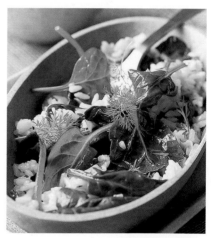

1 Wash the spinach well and drain in a colander. Shake off excess water and shred the leaves coarsely.

2 Heat the olive oil in a large pan and sauté the chopped onion until it is translucent. Add the spinach leaves to the pan and stir for a few minutes to coat with the oil.

3 As soon as the spinach looks wilted, add the lemon juice and water, and bring to the boil. Add the rice and dill, cover and cook gently for about 10 minutes. If it looks too dry, add a little water. Season to taste.

4 Serve hot or at room temperature, placing sprigs of dill over the top.

low-fat comfort food

During the premenstrual countdown, the urge to "pig out" on high-fat foods such as crisps and fries may be immense. This provides the comfort of fries without the harmful fat content.

roasted oven fries

2 large baking potatoes
22ml/1½ tbsp olive oil
5ml/1 tsp fresh herbs such as rosemary and thyme, chopped
scant sprinkling of sea salt (or lemon juice if you are avoiding salt)
low-fat mayonnaise, for dipping

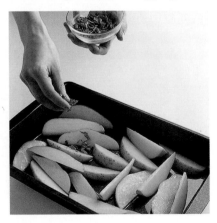

1 Place a roasting pan in the oven and preheat to 240°C/475°F/ Gas 9. Cut the potatoes in half lengthwise, then into thin wedges. When the pan is hot, remove it and put in the oil, potatoes, herbs and sea salt or lemon juice. Toss well to coat the potatoes evenly, spreading them out in a single layer.

2 Roast the potatoes in the oven for 20–25 minutes, turning at least once, until the wedges are golden brown and puffy. Sprinkle with more herbs, if you like, and a little more sea salt or lemon juice to taste. Serve the fries immediately, while hot and crunchy, with low-fat mayonnaise for dipping.

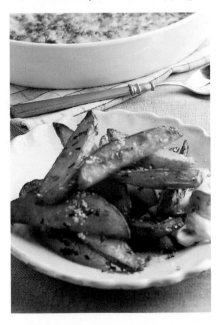

▲ *The hearty crunch and herby taste of these fries satisfies the taste buds.*

10

protein-rich fish

Fish such as tuna can contribute essential protein to your PMS diet regime. Low in saturated fat, it is easy to digest and is a good substitute for red meat, which is best avoided before a period.

seared tuna, bean and noodle Niçoise

Serves 4

2 fresh tuna steaks
175g/6oz fine green beans, trimmed
350g/12oz medium dried egg noodles
225g/8oz halved baby plum tomatoes
3 hard-boiled eggs, quartered
50g/2oz black olives
fresh basil leaves, torn

For the dressing:
90ml/6 tbsp olive oil
30ml/2 tbsp lemon juice
2.5ml/½ tsp Dijon mustard
45ml/3 tbsp chopped parsley

Rinse the tuna steaks. Combine the dressing ingredients in a jar, shake to mix and set aside. Blanch the green beans in boiling water for 4 minutes. Drain, place in a bowl with the noodles, and pour boiling water over to cover. Leave for 5 minutes, then drain and toss the beans and noodles with some of the dressing.

Heat a ridged griddle pan until it is smoking. Place the tuna steaks on the griddle and sear for 1–2 minutes on each side. Remove and immediately slice thinly. Add the tuna, tomatoes, eggs, olives and basil to the beans and noodles; add more dressing to taste.

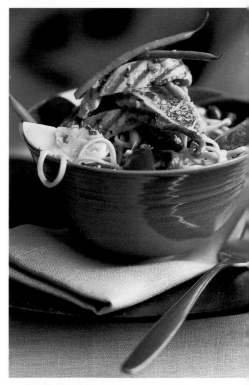

▲ *A perfect substitute for red meat, this tuna dish is low in fat and highly nutritious.*

11 hormone-regulating GLAs

Plant oils containing gamma linolenic acid, or GLA, can ease premenstrual symptoms such as breast tenderness and cramping. Supplements are available in capsule or oil form.

balancing evening primrose

Gamma linolenic acid is an essential fatty acid that aids the production of prostaglandins. These are substances that help to maintain the body's hormonal balance and control the release of the sex hormones, oestrogen and testosterone. Probably the most common source of gamma linolenic acid is evening primrose oil. Taken over time, it has been shown to reduce a range of PMS symptoms, from breast tenderness to joint aches and skin complaints. It also helps to decrease the blood-clotting that can cause cramping. You will begin to feel the benefits of taking evening primrose oil supplements from one to three months after starting. Ask your medical practitioner about dosage.

borage oil

Also called starflower oil, borage oil is the richest source of gamma linolenic acid found in nature, at 22–25 per cent. This proportion is twice that of evening primrose oil. Borage supplements are often combined with evening primrose oil or flax oil, which also contains omega essential fatty acids. For the highest quality, look for capsules of cold-pressed, organic oil.

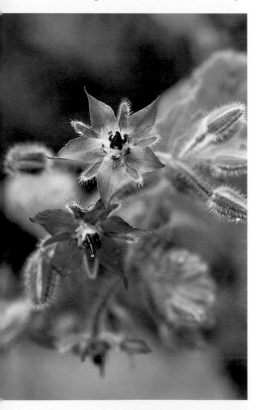

◀ *The borage plant yields an oil that, taken regularly, can help to balance hormones.*

12

vital vitamins C & E

Ensuring that you consume enough vitamins C and E by eating fresh fruits and vegetables will help relieve many PMS conditions. You can use supplements to top up your levels.

easing E

An essential fat-soluble substance, vitamin E is said to ease tenderness in the breasts and decrease the size of fibrous breast lumps before a period. Vitamin E is found in many types of foods, including nuts, seeds such as sunflower and pumpkin, cold-pressed oils, vegetables, spinach, whole grains, wheatgerm oil, asparagus, avocado, beef, seafood and carrots.

For PMS, it may be beneficial to increase the vitamin E in your diet with a daily supplement. Ask your medical practitioner for advice.

get your Cs

A shortage of vitamin C can result in water retention, a lack of energy and poor digestion, so it is a good idea to ensure that you are getting enough prior to and during your period. Also known as ascorbic acid, this vitamin assists with tissue growth, the healing of wounds and burns and the prevention of blood-clotting. Good food sources of vitamin C include

fresh berries, citrus fruits, green leafy vegetables, guavas, tomatoes, melons and peppers. Daily supplements of 500–1,000mg may help to ease the symptoms of PMS.

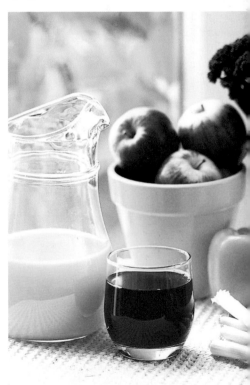

▸ *Citrus fruits and apples are rich sources of vitamin C. Eat whole or drink their juices.*

13

essential B vitamins & B6

Eating food containing a selection of B group vitamins is essential for cell growth, and vitamin B6 in particular may help alleviate many premenstrual symptoms.

B group vitamins

To maintain healthy functioning of the reproductive system, as well as all of the body's other systems, an adequate amount of B vitamins should be consumed.

Nearly all the food groups contain B vitamins. To get a balanced mix, eat foods such as liver, kidney, poultry, fish, eggs, nuts, yeast, cereals, legumes, mushrooms, walnuts, seeds, seafood, vegetables and whole grains. If you also wish to take some multivitamin supplements, these are best taken early in the day, when they provide a physical and mental boost.

vitamin B6

Research has shown that vitamin B6 (pyridoxine) helps to balance female hormones and fight depression. The foods that contain this vitamin include chicken, fish, liver, kidneys, eggs, walnuts and carrots. Taking vitamin supplements of 50–100mg per day may help to relieve PMS symptoms. Be careful not to take over 200mg, as this can cause adverse reactions such as numbness and tingling in the feet and hands.

▼ *Fish is high in B6, while green beans provide important B vitamins.*

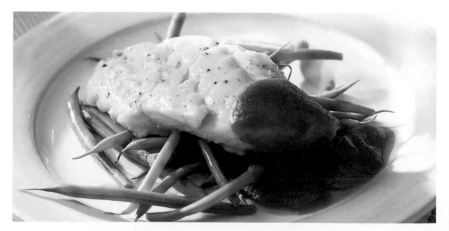

14

craving-reducing magnesium

Magnesium has been shown to reduce cravings for sugar and chocolate. It can also reduce breast tenderness and migraine, two premenstrual symptoms that are suffered by many women.

beneficial mineral

Not only does it reduce the craving for sweets, the mineral magnesium also provides an effective boost to energy levels when you need it most. Magnesium deficiency can lead to tiredness and irritability. It also helps control blood pressure and keeps the heart muscle toned, and it works to help the body absorb calcium, an important mineral for cell function and bone formation.

Recent research in the USA has suggested that magnesium may also play a part in preventing migraines. In the studies, half the women who suffered from menstrual migraine were shown to have a magnesium deficiency at the time of the onset of their headaches.

getting enough

To consume magnesium in your premenstrual diet, choose from a wide selection of magnesium-rich foods, including dairy products, fish, legumes, apples, apricots, avocados, bananas, whole grain cereals, nuts and dark green vegetables. Cocoa is also a source of magnesium, which may be a reason for craving chocolate at this time if there is a deficiency. The recommended supplement dosage is 300–500mg per day, taken only when symptoms are present. Ask your medical practitioner for advice.

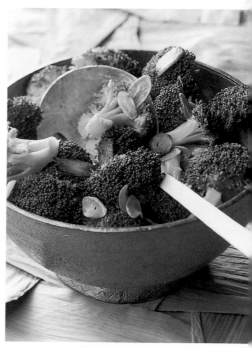

▲ Dark green vegetables such as broccoli are good sources of magnesium.

15 natural diuretics

One of the most aggravating and uncomfortable premenstrual symptoms is water retention, which also triggers other PMS complaints. Herbs and supplements that have a diuretic effect can help.

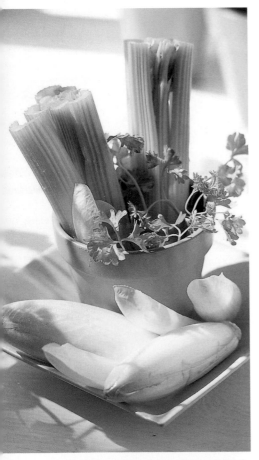

▲ Parsley and celery leaves have a natural diuretic effect on the system.

water weight

Many women experience significant weight gain in the days before a period, due to water retention. A whole host of other symptoms may also stem from it, from swollen breasts and limbs, to dizziness caused by the accumulation of water in the inner ear. Water retention can cause headaches and stuffy sinuses, due to pressure building in the skull, and it is also the cause of premenstrual backaches, stiff muscles and abdominal bloating.

herbal supplements

While there is no way to eradicate water retention totally, it is possible to get temporary relief from herbs and supplements. Chewing parsley or celery leaves can help, and there are many other safe and natural herbal diuretics that are very effective at easing symptoms.

Tablet formulas and tinctures may include any of the following herbs, alone or in combination: boldo, *Uva ursi*, dandelion, juniper, celery and parsley. They are available from most chemists and health food shops. Use them only while symptoms are present.

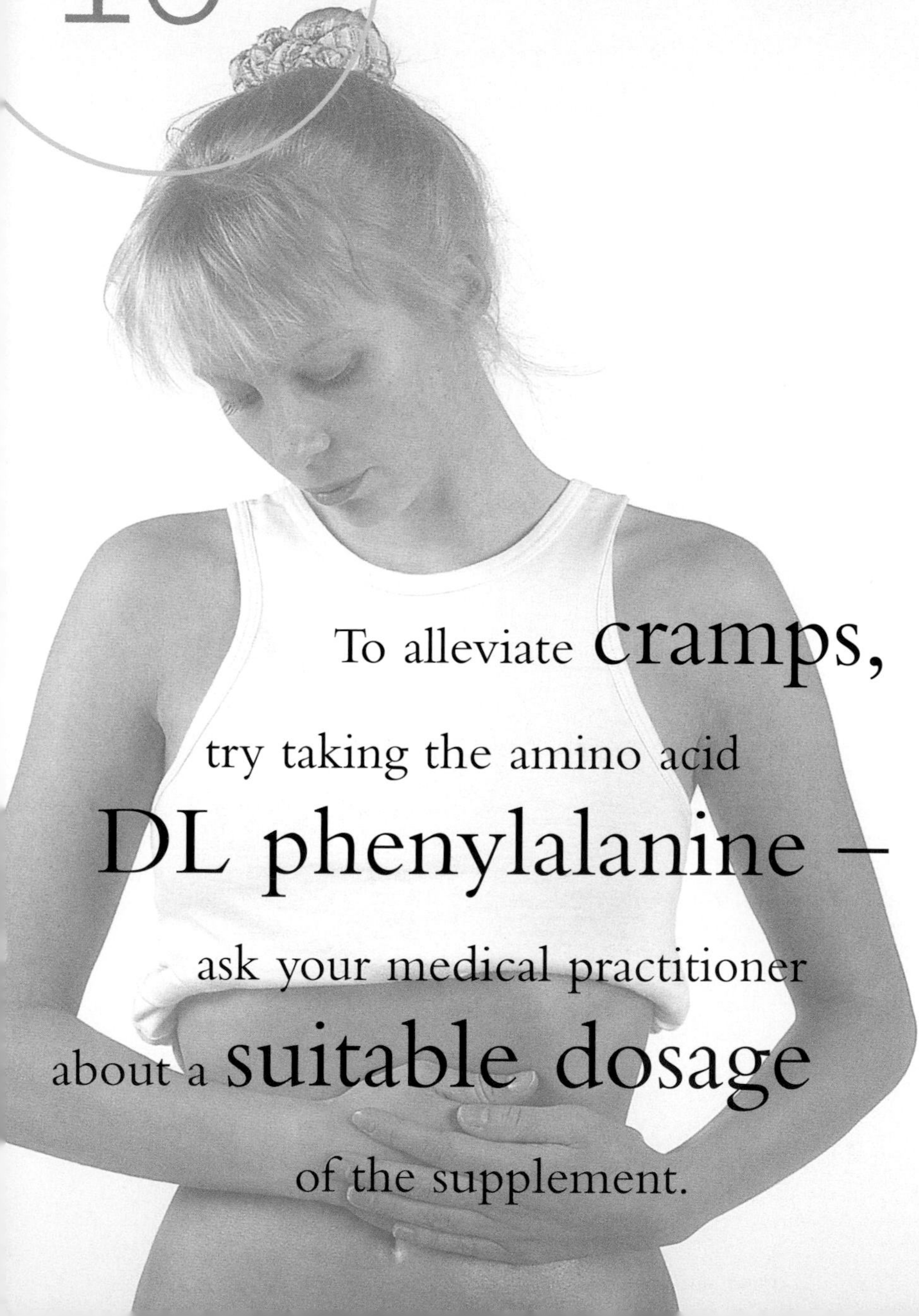

To alleviate cramps,

try taking the amino acid

DL phenylalanine –

ask your medical practitioner

about a suitable dosage

of the supplement.

17 herbal migraine-easers

Unfortunately, headaches and migraines are ailments that are very commonly associated with women's monthly cycles. But herbal remedies may relieve and even work to prevent them.

feverfew relief

With any type of headache, taking a remedy at the first warning sign gives the best results. This is especially crucial with migraines, which can be heralded by symptoms including visual disturbances, a sharp ache at one side of the head, nausea and sensitivity to light, sound and smells.

The herb feverfew, which is a member of the daisy family, contains the active substance parthenolide, which has the effect of inhibiting the body's production of prostaglandins. It therefore reduces the inflammatory reactions they cause, and helps to determine the amount of blood delivered to the tissues. This is significant in migraines, when the narrowing and widening of blood vessels in the brain causes pressure and pain. Take feverfew in the days before your period for prevention, and as early as possible during an attack.

butterburr

Taken regularly, butterburr is said to reduce the occurrence of migraines by about 60 per cent. Clinical trials show that the attacks that occur are less severe, and also of shorter duration. This supplement – along with feverfew – is available from health food stores and internet sites. Ask your healthcare practitioner for the correct dosage.

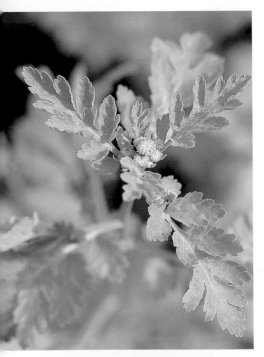

▲ *Feverfew is recommended by many healthcare advisers as a migraine remedy.*

18 relieving nausea & bloating

The days leading up to a period may be beset with digestive problems, from uncomfortable bloating and gassiness, to indigestion and nausea. Natural remedies can help to calm the digestion.

peppermint cure

One of the best and most readily available remedies for digestive upsets is peppermint. Its cooling sensation eliminates abdominal cramps, nausea, gas, bloating and spastic colon. For a digestive after a meal, make a tea from fresh or dried leaves by steeping in boiling water for 5 minutes; or add 1–2 drops peppermint oil to a glass of cold or hot water.

Oil of peppermint capsules are ideal if you are at work or out of the house. Spearmint, with its milder taste, is also beneficial, and can be used in the same way as peppermint. Even chewing strong mint gum can be beneficial, but choose sugar-free varieties to prevent tooth decay.

comforting ginger

A root used for thousands of years in China, ginger is very effective in soothing irritation of the intestinal membranes and aiding digestion. To use fresh ginger, simply slice a piece of root thinly and place two or three slices in a cup. Pour on boiling water and allow to steep for 5 minutes. Add a teaspoon of honey to sweeten if desired, and drink. Powdered ginger may also be used.

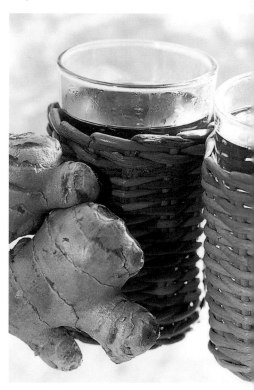

▸ *Fresh ginger slices can be infused in boiling water to make a delicious, fragrant digestive that brings instant relief.*

19 natural progesterone

Wild yam extract has been used for centuries in many cultures for its natural progesterone content. It can be used to treat a whole host of ailments, including premenstrual symptoms.

hormone imbalance

As the body ages, its production of progesterone – a hormone produced by the ovaries and also, to a lesser extent, by the adrenal glands – declines dramatically, leading to hormonal imbalances caused by an excess of oestrogen. These imbalances can lead to increased premenstrual symptoms, including water retention, variations in blood sugar levels (leading to mood and energy dips), depression and sleep disturbances.

wild yam extract

Natural progesterone creams made from plants such as wild yam can help normalize blood sugar levels, help the body use fat for energy, and clear up premenstrual acne and skin redness. They also have a natural diuretic and anti-depressant effect, and have been said to help prevent breast and endometrial cancers.

Progesterone cream is applied by rubbing it into the soft skin on the inner thigh, upper inner arm, chest or behind the knees. For PMS symptoms, 2.5ml/½ tsp is normally used twice daily for 21 days, stopping for seven days at the beginning of your cycle. Ask your healthcare practitioner for more information.

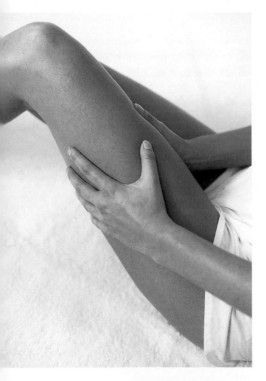

◂ *Progesterone cream is rubbed into the skin at soft tissue spots, where it is easily absorbed by the body.*

20 protective calcium

Calcium is an essential nutrient for women; it has been shown to be helpful in preventing and relieving premenstrual symptoms, and is important in the prevention of osteoporosis.

multiple relief

According to recent research, taking adequate calcium can help to reduce the physical and emotional effects of PMS by up to 50 per cent. Depression, mood swings, breast tenderness and abdominal and leg cramps may be relieved by ensuring that you eat enough foods containing calcium. Few people actually hit the recommended target of 1,000mg of calcium per day; some estimates indicate that the average woman manages only 500–700mg a day. So a supplement may be beneficial.

daily dose

Doctors recommend that women of child-bearing age should try to eat from a selection of dairy products such as milk, yogurt and cheese, and should also eat leafy green vegetables such as spinach, not just when PMS symptoms are present, but at all times of the month.

Try to work out how much calcium you get through your diet. If you think you have a shortfall, it may be a good idea to boost the amount to 1,000–1,200mg by taking a daily supplement of calcium carbonate.

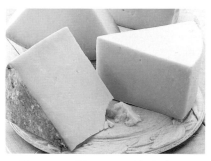

▲ Cheese provides a concentrated amount of calcium. Choose low-fat varieties.

▶ Drinking semi-skimmed or skimmed milk is a good way to top up your calcium level.

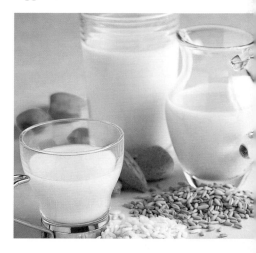

21

yoga for PMS

Excellent exercises at any time of the month, certain yoga postures – or asanas – can help to alleviate symptoms such as cramps, irregularity, backache, muscle ache and emotional tension.

wide-angled seated pose

On one or two folded blankets, sit with your back straight against a wall and arms at your sides. Spread your legs apart, as wide as possible. Keep the fronts of the legs facing the ceiling and the feet upright. Straighten the knees, then pull the thigh muscles back towards the groin. Draw up the trunk to extend the spine and open up the chest. Be sure to breathe evenly throughout. Stay in this position for 2–3 minutes, then release.

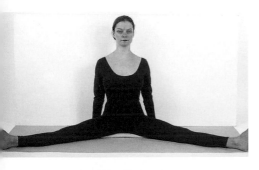

CAUTION:
You should not practise yoga poses during menstruation because they may interfere with the natural flow of blood.

half-lotus forward bend

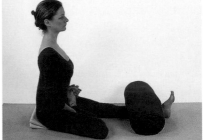

1 On a folded blanket, sit with your back straight and shoulders relaxed, with arms at your sides. Bend the right leg and place the foot on top of the left thigh, in the groin. Place a bolster on the left shin.

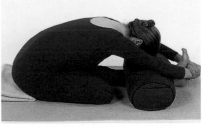

2 Bend forward and hold the left foot, resting your head on the bolster. Stay in this position for 30–40 seconds, then repeat on the other side.

22 toning Pilates

Pilates is a system of exercise that aids muscle flexibility. It tones the girdle of muscles in the abdomen, strengthening the back and lessening the incidence of premenstrual backache.

the method

The Pilates Method was developed by Joseph Pilates over 70 years ago, and many variations of the exercise system have evolved since. Some forms are performed on specially designed exercise equipment, but many are carried out on the floor, using only a simple mat.

Using a series of controlled movements and breathing, Pilates exercises are designed to strengthen the deep postural muscles, building a "girdle of muscles" around the torso that protects your back from injury, aches and pains. The gentle movement makes for a refreshing workout that tones the whole body, while also improving the circulation, respiratory and lymphatic systems.

receiving instruction

Look for classes conducted by a qualified instructor at your local gym or leisure centre. Light, comfortable clothing is required, and the exercises are usually performed in bare feet or socks. Step-by-step Pilates videos are also available: these are good if you want to work at your own pace, or wish to do only some of the stretches to relieve PMS backache.

▼ *Pilates strengthens abdominal muscles.*

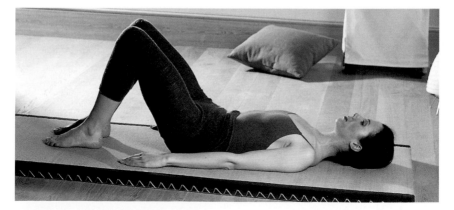

23 stress-alleviating aerobics

When you're feeling anxious or down in the days before your period, doing an aerobic activity of your choice is one of the best ways to relieve stress and lift depression.

PMS specialists maintain that aerobic exercise, which raises the heart rate and is fuelled by oxygen, is essential for staying mentally and physically healthy, especially if you become frustrated, irritated and angry during the last two weeks of your cycle.

You need not attend a formal aerobics class: any activity that works up a sweat is aerobic. If you work sitting in an office all day, running up and down the stairs for a few minutes will make you feel better. Walking all or part of the way to and from work also helps you to wind down. Our bodies were designed to move, not to sit at a desk all day. Exercise uses up the hormone adrenaline that is produced when we become tense.

slow steps

If you have not exercised for a while, you may want to start by taking a leisurely 20-minute stroll during your lunch break, or getting out your bicycle after dinner and taking a tour of the neighbourhood with a friend. These gentle activities are a good choice when PMS symptoms such as tender breasts and cramps occur.

On the days that you feel more vigorous – possibly around ovulation, about 14 days before your period begins – tennis, badminton, dancing, jogging and running can all release tension. Whichever exercise you choose, aim to do a session of about 30 minutes at least three times a week.

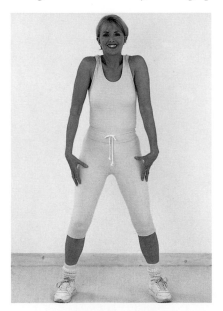

◀ *Stretching the muscles before aerobic activity warms them and prevents injury.*

24
muscle fatigue relievers

Aching muscles – especially in the limbs – are a very common premenstrual symptom. These simple stretches will help to prevent the build-up of muscle tension.

calf stretch

Sit on the floor with one leg stretched out in front of you. Lean forward and grasp your foot with your hand. Pull your foot gently towards you, feeling the tightness in the calf. Hold for 30 seconds. If you cannot hold the foot in this position, try doing this stretch with the leg slightly bent. Repeat the exercise with the other leg.

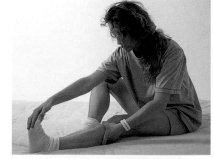

finger pulls

Squeeze a finger joint of one hand between the first finger and thumb of the other hand. Hold the base of the finger and then pull the finger gently, sliding your grip up to the top in a continuous movement. Repeat the exercise with all the fingers and thumbs of each hand.

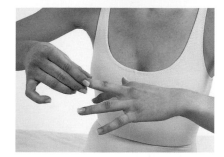

hamstring stretch

Lie down flat on the floor or exercise mat. Raise one leg and bend the other knee. Stretch the muscle in the raised leg by pulling it gently towards your chest. Hold for 20 seconds. Relax, then repeat with the other leg.

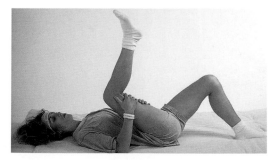

25 abdominal tension easer

Premenstrual emotional stress can lead to tension being stored in the abdominal area. These two exercises can help to loosen up the muscles, helping you to relax and breathe more deeply.

sideways bends

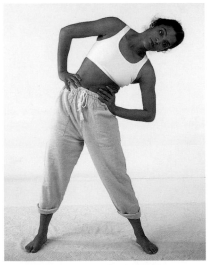

1 Stand with your feet apart and your hands on your hips. Bend over to one side, keeping your head in line with your torso – do not twist the body.

2 Slowly return to an upright position, then bend to the other side. Repeat on each side eight times. Do not bend further than is comfortable. Your flexibility should improve as you get used to the movement.

abdominal moves

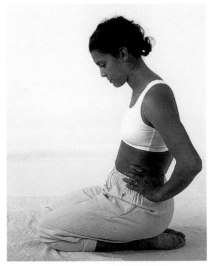

1 Sit cross-legged or kneel in a comfortable position, and place your hands on your waist or thighs. Let your breath out completely.

2 Without inhaling, pull in your abdomen as far as you can, then let it "snap" in and out up to five times before you take a breath. Relax for a few moments, then repeat the sequence three times.

Use the support of comforting

water to stretch fatigued

muscles and tissues

before your period – try

swimming,
aqua aerobics or
water jogging.

27

pine & rosemary back rub

Premenstrual tension can leave your neck and back aching and sore. This refreshing mixture, used in conjunction with massage from your partner or a friend, will bring you lasting relief.

Good for muscular aches and stiffness, marjoram and rosemary are both effective treatments, while invigorating oil of pine seeps deep into muscle tissue to provide relief from pain; it also relieves fatigue. You can ask your partner to massage the oil into tense areas, or use self-massage to work it into your neck and upper back.

pine, rosemary and marjoram rub

15ml/1 tbsp safflower, wheatgerm, jojoba or other carrier oil
1 drop pine essential oil
2 drops rosemary essential oil
2 drops marjoram essential oil

Wash and dry your hands, and make sure that the utensils are clean and dry. Measure the carrier oil into a small bowl. Add the pine, rosemary and marjoram oils, one drop at a time. Mix gently with a clean cocktail stick (toothpick).

> **CAUTION:**
> If you have sensitive skin, make a test mix with just one drop of essential oil to 20ml/4 tsp carrier oil and apply to a small area of skin before using for a full massage.

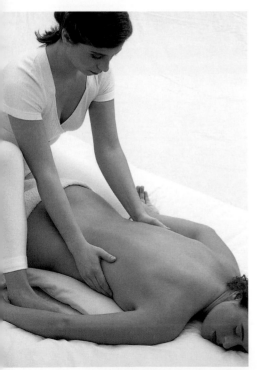

◀ *A relaxing and deep back rub using an essential oil mixture will calm frayed nerves as well as soothing your body.*

28 hormone-balancing bath oil

An increase of premenstrual oestrogen can lead to a range of complaints. This relaxing bath mix uses essences that may help to normalize hormonal secretions, easing the onset of symptoms.

Renowned for their beneficial effect on the female reproductive system, clary sage and naiouli relax cramped muscles, while cypress helps ovarian problems. Use this bath oil for 10–12 days before the start of your period.

clary sage, naiouli and cypress bath
15ml/1 tbsp almond or other
    carrier oil
1 drop clary sage essential oil
2 drops naiouli essential oil
1 drop cypress essential oil

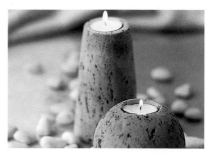

▲ Setting the mood by lighting candles can help bring you into a state of relaxing calm.

Run a very warm bath, but don't make the water too hot. Add the essential oils to the carrier oil in a small bowl and mix. Pour into the bath and swirl the water to distribute the oil. You may want to light candles and play soft music to help you wind down. Climb in and relax for not more than 15–20 minutes.

CAUTION:
Clary sage should not be used if you suspect you may be pregnant. Extensive usage can cause problems with those taking the contraceptive pill or hormone replacement therapy (HRT).

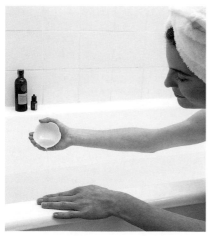

▲ Breathe deeply to experience the full healing effect of the essential oils.

29

crampbark & rosemary abdomen compress

Sharp abdominal pain just before and during periods is due to the contraction of the womb muscles, which reduces blood flow. This hot compress acts to increase blood circulation.

pain-relieving abdomen compress
Crampbark is a herb that works to reduce spasm in the muscles, while rosemary, which is commonly grown in domestic gardens, is a circulatory stimulant that is particularly effective for treating conditions of the womb and the head.

Combining the fresh or dried herbs with the action of heat makes this compress an effective alternative to taking analgesic drugs, providing immediate relief from abdominal pain with no side effects.

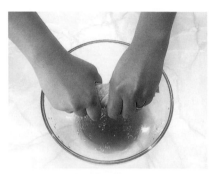

2 Soak a clean cotton cloth or cotton bandage in the liquid. Wring out when the cloth or bandage is cool enough to handle.

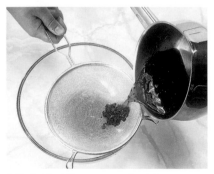

1 Boil 10ml/2 tsp crampbark in 600ml/1 pint/2½ cups water for 10–15 minutes. Add 10ml/2 tsp dried rosemary, or 15ml/3 tsp fresh leaves. Leave for 15 minutes, then strain.

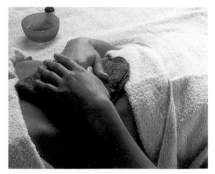

3 Lie down in a comfortable, warm place, lay the hot compress over your abdomen and relax for at least 10 minutes while the soothing properties of the herbs take effect.

30 migraine easer

A painful and debilitating complaint, migraine may be triggered by hormonal changes around menstruation. This remedy can help, but do not use clary sage if you think you may be pregnant.

early action

Many women experience an "aura", seeing a light halo around objects, the day before a migraine attack begins. Some sufferers have a heightened sensitivity to smell. At the earliest sign of a migraine, you can try using this aromatherapy treatment. Add 2 drops rosemary, 1 drop clary sage and 1 drop marjoram to 15ml/1 tbsp of a light carrier oil such as sweet almond or jojoba. Mix the oils together, then rub a small quantity of the oil between the fingers to warm it.

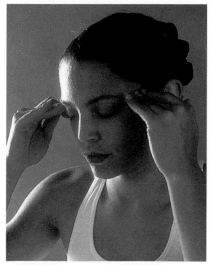

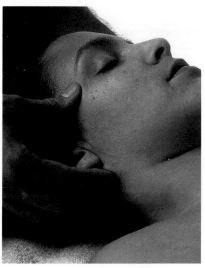

1 Self-massage can be effective. Begin by gently massaging the temples with the oil, using small circular movements. Move the fingers up to massage the forehead and then bring them back to the temples.

2 A gentle head massage from a partner can be even more beneficial. Ask them to massage a small amount of oil into your temples and forehead, then gently work into the hairline and the back of the neck.

31

eucalyptus & lemon inhalation

Minor yet annoying respiratory and sinus problems are common PMS symptoms. An inhalation that uses natural menthol and purifying lemon can help you to breathe more easily.

During the week leading up to their period, many women experience an annoying catarrh at the back of their throat, or suffer from stuffed sinuses. The vocal cords may also become tight, making life more difficult for speakers and singers. As well as drinking plenty of water, using a steam inhalation moistens and warms the membranes; adding essential oils helps to open and relax the airways. Eucalyptus is particularly helpful for the sinuses, chest and nose, and lemon has a cleansing effect.

easy breathing inhalation
Boil a kettle and pour the hot water into a wide bowl. Add 3 drops eucalyptus essential oil and 2 drops lemon essential oil; you could try using 1–2 more drops for a stronger effect. Tilt your head over the bowl and inhale deeply for 2–3 minutes. Keep a comfortable distance away from the steam as it can burn the skin.

▾ *Steam inhalations can be a fast and effective way to provide immediate relief from minor respiratory complaints.*

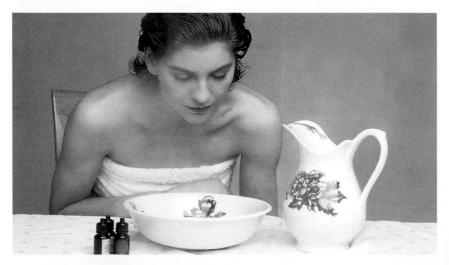

32

calming incenses & oils

Many people find the burning of incense resin or essential oils very soothing during times of premenstrual stress, either when doing meditation or simply while relaxing.

frankincense and myrrh

Used for centuries in religious ceremonies and as a meditation aid, frankincense deepens and slows the breath. It dispels nervous tension and fear, and is useful for painful periods. Myrrh has also been used since ancient times; it has antiseptic and healing qualities that cleanse the air and calm the spirits. Add 2 drops frankincense and 2 drops myrrh essential oils to water in the bowl of an oil burner. Alternatively, burn nuggets of both resins in a charcoal burner, or use incense sticks.

orange, neroli and benzoin

Another calming combination to try is neroli, benzoin and orange peel. Neroli soothes the nerves with its hypnotic and euphoric effect, and can bestow a sense of peace during times of premenstrual tension, anxiety and low self-confidence. Benzoin is soothing for temporary emotional turbulence, such as that caused by pre-period mood swings. It helps you to let go of worries and quells feelings of depression. The addition of orange gives a lift to the senses and relieves exhaustion. For an aromatherapy mix, add 2 drops neroli, 2 drops benzoin and 2 drops orange essential oils to water in the bowl of an oil burner.

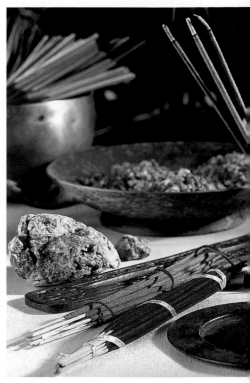

▲ *Burning frankincense and myrrh can help release tension and aid meditation.*

33 rose & jasmine soother

The days leading up to a period may be fraught with frustrated and angry feelings. This oil blend can help if you start to feel tense and critical of family, friends and colleagues.

The abdomen is the "seat of the emotions" – tension may build and be stored here, causing irritation, especially before menstruation. This calming abdominal rub can be used as a salve to calm frayed nerves. The beautiful scents of rose and jasmine are both uplifting and soothing to the nervous system.

rose and jasmine soother

In a bowl or bottle, add 3 drops of rose essential oil and 3 drops jasmine essential oil to 75ml/5 tbsp of carrier oil such as almond to make up a massage oil; stir or shake to disperse.

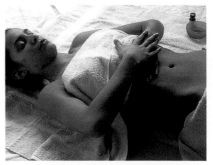

2 Move your hands in a clockwise direction, trying to keep the muscles relaxed the whole time. Breathe deeply to get the benefit of the scent.

ROSE

The rose has been prized throughout history for its restorative properties, including treatment of irregular and painful periods, headaches, insomnia, depression and stomach upsets of an emotional origin.

JASMINE

The strong smell of jasmine – which has been described as "the scent of angels" – is good for general PMS complaints and painful periods. It promotes feelings of optimism, euphoria and confidence.

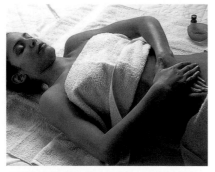

1 Using a little of the oil in your palms, slowly and firmly rub the abdomen with your hands.

The **chaste tree** berry

has been known to ease general

PMS symptoms.

For best effect, take drops of the

tincture two or three times

daily during the week before

menstruation.

35 lower back relaxer

The lumbar area of the back, where it curves towards the pelvis, is a common premenstrual hot spot. A massage from your partner will do much to alleviate discomfort and pain.

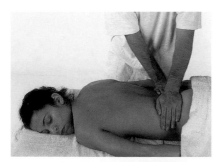

1 Find somewhere comfortable for your partner to lie for the treatment. Standing or kneeling to the side, place your hands on the opposite side of your partner's back and pull them toward you firmly. Work down the back to the base of the spine, always keeping in mind the comfort of the person you are massaging.

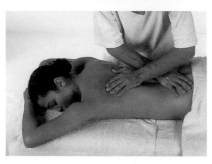

2 Overlap the hands to create an effect similar to bandaging, but ensure that you do this with a soothing, caressing motion. Because this can be a sensitive and painful area at this time of the month, ask your partner how hard she would like the pressure to be and adjust your movements as necessary.

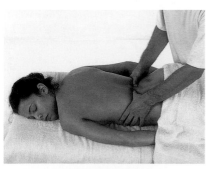

3 Using your thumbs, make circling movements over the lower back. Use a steady, even pressure, leaning with your body, but do not press on the spine because this might cause discomfort and pain. Continue this movement for approximately 5 minutes, then repeat step 2, but use lighter movements in order to end the massage.

36 fluid retention reducer

Many women experience uncomfortable water retention during the last two weeks of their cycle. This massage will help release water from cells in the thighs and legs.

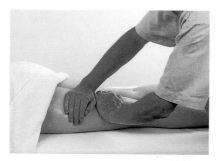

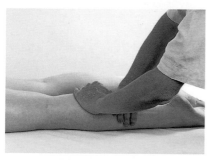

thigh and leg massage

1 In order to improve someone's circulation, warm a little massage oil in the palms of your hands, then oil the legs. Place both hands on the thigh and stroke upward to the buttocks a few times. Use light but steady sweeping movements, hand-over-hand.

2 Move hands down to the lower leg and stroke up to the back of the knee a few times. Repeat steps 1 and 2 on the other leg, remembering always to stroke upward toward the heart.

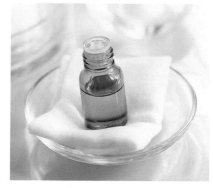

▲ *Lemon oil is an excellent essential oil for reducing water retention. Use a little at first to check whether your skin is sensitive to it.*

THERAPEUTIC OILS
The essential oil from the juniper berry has a diuretic effect, so for massage you can add 2 drops to 30ml/2 tbsp carrier oil. Other oils to try include grapefruit, geranium and lemon oil. Use citrus oils sparingly until you are sure that your skin is not sensitive to them.

37 abdomen massage

A gentle massage from a partner or friend can help relieve premenstrual cramping and discomfort in the abdominal region. Do not use this massage after a heavy meal.

A drop or two of peppermint or spearmint oil added to a tablespoon of carrier oil – such as grapeseed or sunflower – will add a soothing, cool dimension to this massage. The essential oils of the mint family contain menthol, which is a natural digestive that can be helpful when used externally as well as internally.

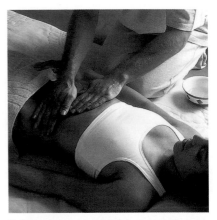

2 Adjust the depth of pressure to your partner's comfort level. If it is increased slowly and gradually, deeper pressure can be very relaxing, but you should not overdo it.

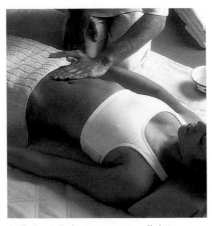

1 Rub a little massage oil into your hands to warm it. On the abdomen, use very slow circling movements in a clockwise direction, to aid the digestive process. Make sure your partner feels comfortable with this movement and is relaxed.

> **ABDOMINAL PAIN**
> Regular full-body massage using recommended essential oils, such as chamomile, clary sage, hops, lavender, marjoram, rose and rosemary, can help to alleviate period pains. However, severe pain should always be investigated by a medical practitioner, as it may indicate a gynaecological disorder.

38 helpful homeopathy

Many women are prone to premenstrual mood swings and pain. Homeopathy treatments, whereby tiny amounts of plant, mineral or animal substances are taken, can help.

Homeopathy is a holistic therapy based on the principle of "like cures like". Formulated by Samuel Hahnemann in the 19th century, it works on the premise that infinitesimally small amounts of a substance which, in a healthy person, would produce symptoms of a particular complaint, will stimulate the immune system of a sufferer to combat that same complaint. A range of remedies, taken singly or together, can help ease PMS symptoms.

emotional rescue

Along with moodiness, some women are beset with symptoms of depression, anger and weepiness, even as much as a week or more before the flow begins. *Pulsatilla* is an excellent remedy if weeping and the feeling of neediness are prominent. *Sepia* can be used where there is anger and exhaustion, and can even lessen feelings of indifference to your family. For extreme symptoms of violent anger and jealousy, *Lachesis* is helpful.

▸ Consult a qualified practitioner for advice on homeopathic treatments for PMS.

period pain aid

For cramping pains that respond to warmth (a hot water bottle, for example) and make you want to curl up, *Mag phos* should provide some relief. For very severe pains with bad cramping, *Viburnum opulus* is a powerful painkiller.

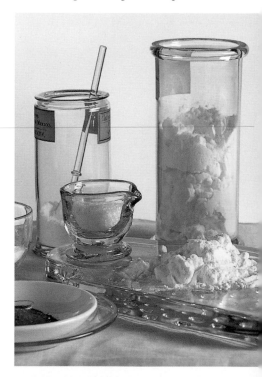

Find a quiet spot, and sit with your hands resting lightly on your lap.

Close your eyes and draw in a deep breath from the bottom of your lungs, counting to ten. Slowly release on another count of ten.

40 relieving reflexology

Reflexology works on the premise that reflex points on the feet, hands and head correspond to other areas of the body. It can help ease PMS symptoms such as cramps and aching breasts.

menstrual cramps

Applying pressure with the thumb and fingers to the areas marked on the feet in the photographs can provide relief for abdominal cramps around the time of menstruation.

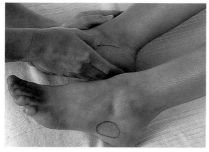

1 Work the lower spine for nerves to the uterus.

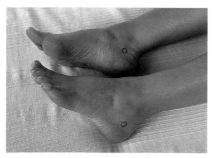

2 Next, work the uterus reflex on the sides of the heels.

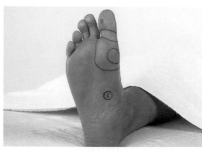

3 Finally, work the glands on one foot and repeat on the other.

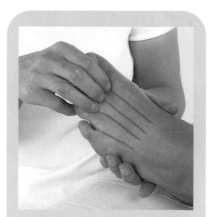

TENDER BREASTS
To soothe painful or tender breasts, fingerwalk up the "chest" area, marked on top of the foot, with three fingers together.

healing Reiki

A quick and subtle treatment, Reiki works on the premise that the practitioner helps the healing flow of energy in you, the recipient, assisting your own body and emotions to heal themselves.

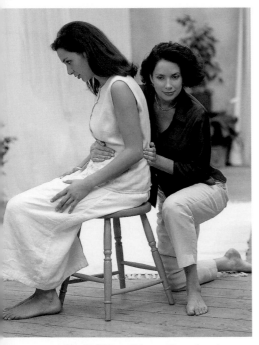

▲ The Reiki practitioner places hands directly on your body to direct energy flow.

power over pain

Perhaps Reiki's greatest gift is the empowerment of individuals to take responsibility for themselves and their own healing. Reiki energy can be so fast-acting, yet so subtle, that some

ailments can fade away almost imperceptibly, together with the emotional triggers that may have been behind them. When considering Reiki treatment for premenstrual symptoms, it is best to make an appointment with a qualified Reiki practitioner. Many practitioners are happy to teach you self-treatment techniques. Some also practise "distance Reiki" – a healing flow of energy sent to you without your having to be in the healer's presence.

menstrual pain

In Reiki healing for menstrual pain, the practitioner will ask you to sit down or perhaps to stretch out on a sofa. She will then place one hand on your lower stomach and the other on the lower back, for relief from pain and cramping. This will lighten and relieve the surrounding area, including the thighs.

One philosophy associated with Reiki treatment is that women can use this time to celebrate female unity and the expression of female energy, rather than view their pain as a purely negative thing.

42

emotion-balancing crystals

Period pain and menstrual cramps are often made worse by physical and emotional tension restricting the body's natural energy flow. Crystals can help to redress the balance.

mood-adjusting moonstones

In crystal therapy, moonstones, whether natural, tumbled or gem-polished, are said to be the ideal stones for women to wear, according to ancient Indian Ayurvedic texts. Moonstone is helpful in balancing and relaxing emotional states. It also has beneficial effects on all fluid systems in the body, and eases tension in the abdominal area.

A healing pattern of five moonstones amplifies the relaxing and healing potential of the stones. Place one moonstone at the top of your head, one on the front of each shoulder by the armpit and one resting on each hip.

chakra-opening opals

Dark opal has similar qualities to those of the moonstone, though it acts mainly on the first chakra – the energy centre that balances the sense of "self" – and the second chakra, the base of the sexual organs and the emotions, where it can often ease menstrual cramps in a very short time. Place a small piece of opal in a hip or trouser pocket.

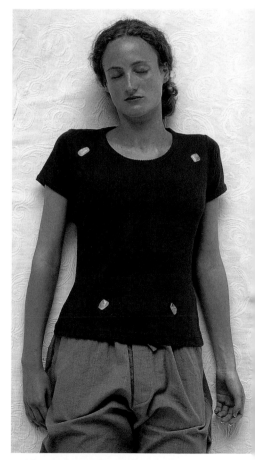

▲ *Moonstones and opals help to open up the chakras, assisting emotional healing.*

43 dealing with moodiness

Many women become susceptible to mood swings and depression in the week before a period, but there are a number of positive measures you can take to give yourself a lift.

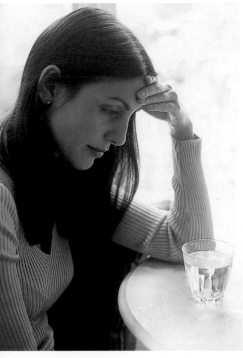

▲ *If you can control your thoughts, you can steer your mood into a more positive vein.*

take time out

You think you're having a great day, then suddenly someone says the wrong thing and you snap. From anger and frustration to anxiety and panic, hormones can play havoc with the moods and emotions. First of all, stop and remind yourself what time of the month it is, and give yourself a little slack. It's better not to take your frustrations out on others, so if you need a few minutes on your own, make your excuses and go for a walk, or sit and meditate in a quiet place. Take a deep breath and try to reach your "centre" – the true you beyond turbulent emotions or obsessive thoughts. But if you are feeling seriously depressed or out of control, talk to your doctor or a counsellor – don't suffer in silence.

make laughter essential

PMS can make some women feel stressed or unable to cope. One of the best ways of dealing with these feelings is to make sure you have a good laugh every day. Laughter raises the level of endorphins, the body's "feel good" substances. Sharing a few jokes with friends is a good way to dissipate negativity, as is watching a funny film or television show. Stepping back and laughing at your own dramas is excellent medicine.

44 enhancing relationships

Many women experience an increase in libido before or during their periods. Instead of letting the energy lead to frustration, you can use this time to explore your sexuality with your partner.

Emotions and sexual urges can run high from the time of ovulation through to your period. This provides a good opportunity to try new techniques and ways of lovemaking with your partner. You could start by giving each other an intimate massage, or sharing a bath. Perhaps you could share sexual thoughts and fantasies, then decide which ones to act out. Create a sensual atmosphere by lighting candles, sharing wine and shutting out the rest of the world.

▾ *Intimacy can lead you both to explore your depth of feeling for each other.*

beyond the physical
As well as reading books on sexual technique, it can be enlightening to explore different approaches to sex, such as the holistic view of lovemaking of Tantric philosophy. This school of thought evolved in ancient India and Tibet about 5,000 years ago. Today it is practised by those who want to enjoy greater intimacy of mind, body and spirit with their partner. Tantra sees a sexual relationship not only as the physical union of two people, but a re-enactment of the divine principle of union that governs the whole of existence.

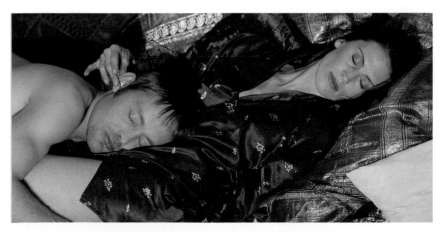

45 creative time out

For women of many cultures around the world, menstruation is seen as a time to celebrate their womanhood and the natural cycle of life, not as a time to be dreaded or ignored.

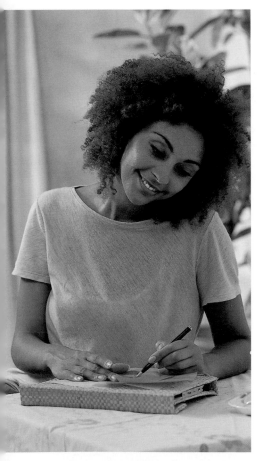

▲ *Many women use the "down time" in their natural cycles to reflect and create.*

a place away

Traditionally, among tribal peoples such as Native North Americans, a special menstrual hut was built so that a woman could go and be on her own to gather her thoughts, and find ideas through dreams and meditation. When she emerged from this "moontime", as it is sometimes called, it would be with songs, stories and insights into future endeavours. In such cultures it is believed that, just as the moon waxes and wanes, a woman reflects the changes in nature in her monthly cycle, and she is treasured for being this way.

meaningful moontime

You can make this time of every month a positive pathway to personal growth and change. By taking time to rest and reflect, instead of fighting the urge to slow down, you may be surprised by the clarity of the new ideas that surface. Indulge in your favourite pursuit or hobby, and give yourself room just to "be" with it – whether it is painting, music, cooking, astronomy, or devising a new system for your line of work.

46

soothing meditation

Meditation can help to bring body and mind into a state of harmony, allowing you to see your world in perspective. This meditation uses the clarity and depth of water imagery to focus the mind.

the well

You find yourself standing near the edge of a pond, looking down into the clear, cool water, gazing at goldfish, red and gold, black and silver, swimming so easily . . . gliding effortlessly in and out of the pondweed and around the lily pads. Your mind becomes deeply relaxed. You notice that the centre of the pond is very, very deep. It could be the top of a disused well . . . You take a silver coin and toss it into the very centre of the pond . . . then watch as it swivels down through the water. Ripples form, but you just watch the coin as it drifts and sinks, deeper and deeper through the clear water . . . Sometimes it seems to disappear as it turns on edge; at other times a face of the coin catches the sunlight and flashes through the water . . . twisting and turning on its way down . . .

Finally, it comes to rest at the bottom of the pond, lying on a cushion of soft brown mud . . . And you feel as still and undisturbed as the coin . . . as still, cool and motionless as the water, enjoying the feeling of inner peace and utter tranquillity.

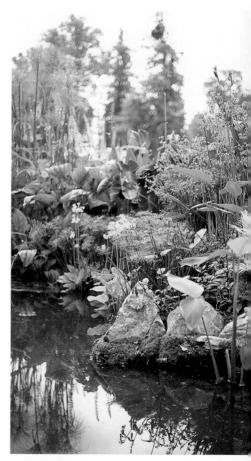

▲ *Gazing into a still pond can help you to still your mind for meditation.*

moon cycles

The moon has been linked with women and the female reproductive cycle from the earliest times. Most moon deities, such as the Greek Artemis and her Roman counterpart Diana, are female.

Many ancient civilizations venerated the moon because they saw how she influenced the germination and growth of crops, and how she also matched the average female menstrual cycle of 28–30 days. Some ancient cultures worshipped several moon goddesses, who represented the

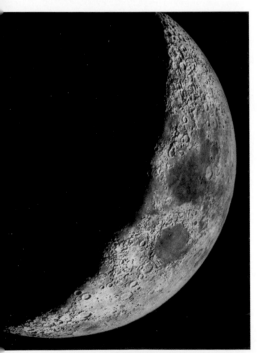

different phases of the moon. The Greeks, for example, honoured Artemis as the new moon, Selene as the full moon and Hecate as the waning and dark moon.

To understand your place in the fertility cycle of nature, it can help to study the moon lore of different cultures and see how these concepts can be related to the energy flow of your own monthly cycle.

female synchronicity
It is a well-known phenomenon that the menstrual cycles of women who live in close proximity to each other – whether flatmates, colleagues, mother and daughters, sisters or friends – tend to synchronize so that their periods start at the same time. This can happen surprisingly quickly, so if you start a new job or get a new flatmate, your menstrual start days may shift over one or two months. One theory is that the woman with the most healthy immune system leads.

◄ *The moon and her cycles have always been linked with women's cycles, both physically and spiritually.*

48

planning ahead

By keeping a chart of premenstrual symptoms, both physical and emotional, you will be able to get an overview of the impact they have on your life, thus allowing you to plan ahead.

Apart from illustrating the rhythm of your life, compiling a chart will help you plan tasks for days of the month when you are feeling more energetic. It will help you to anticipate possible bouts of moodiness and frustration, and signal when you should start taking preventive supplements for these symptoms as well as maladies such as headaches and menstrual cramps.

	J	F	M	A	M	J	J	A	S	O	N	D
1												
2												
3												
4												
5												
6												
7												
8												
9												
10												
11												
12												
13												
14												
15												
16												
17												
18												
19												
20												
21												
22												
23												
24												
25												
26												
27												
28												
29												
30												
31												

Use this simple key to record symptoms, along with "M" for menstruation days.

D = Depression
T = Tearfulness
I = Irritability
S = Sleep disturbance
F = Fatigue
A = Abdominal cramps
H = Headache
J = Joint stiffness
B = Bloating
G = General aches/backache
C = Food cravings
W = Weight gain

49

sleep therapy

Especially during your period, which places special demands on your body, getting a good night's sleep is essential if you are to feel your best throughout the day.

setting the sleep scene

Make sure that your bedroom environment is quiet, pleasant, comfortable and airy. A woman's body temperature normally rises slightly before her period, so wear a lighter nightgown. If you are prone to premenstrual insomnia, try a sedative herbal infusion, such as chamomile or valerian tea, or a hot milky drink, an hour before going to bed. Fresh bedlinen and sprigs of fragrant lavender on your bedside table will help ease you into slumber.

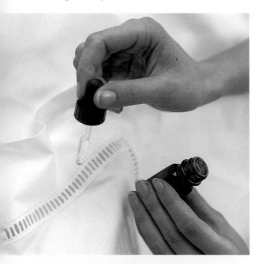

calming mood

Sometimes it is difficult to sleep due to excessive emotions such as fear, depression or anxiety, caused by hormonal changes. Meditation techniques – such as surrounding yourself with a healing colour or visualizing a spiritual protector – can help quell your jumpy nerves. Try not to watch disturbing or violent television shows or read thrillers before going to sleep – these can enter your thought stream unawares and add to, or actually create, anxiety. Instead, read poetry or "light" stories, and listen to soothing music.

sweet dreams

Many women experience vivid and colourful dreams around their periods. Enjoy these by writing down the plots, along with inspiring images or ideas. Pay particular attention to people in your dreams: you could gain special insights about friends and family members, as telepathy can be strong at this time of the month.

◀ *Scent your bedlinen with a few drops of soothing lavender essential oil.*

50

confidence boosters

PMS can make you very self-critical, and you may suffer from temporary low self-esteem. Reminding yourself of achievements and spending time with friends can serve to boost your confidence.

positive affirmations

Make a list of your achievements and attributes you are proud of, and stick it on a mirror or the refrigerator as a reminder of why you are lovable, competent, fun to be with and attractive. For example, your list could include affirmations such as: "I am a lovable person", "I am very good at painting or cooking", "My work colleagues hold me in great esteem", "I am a wonderful partner/mother/ friend", "I am physically beautiful/ have great legs/attractive eyes".

You can also remind yourself, "I may be feeling clumsy and lethargic at the moment, but this is natural and I accept it. In five days I will be my energetic self again."

enjoyable activities

Another way to increase your confidence when you're feeling low is to make time to do something you enjoy every day. Tell yourself that you are worth it, even if you are busy. Drop your chores, work or other responsibilities for an hour and do something you love doing – it is guaranteed to boost your spirits.

Make sure you also spend time talking with friends and family. Ask for the reassurance and physical contact – such as hugs – that you need. They will be happy to help out, and this will enable them to ask for support in turn when they need it.

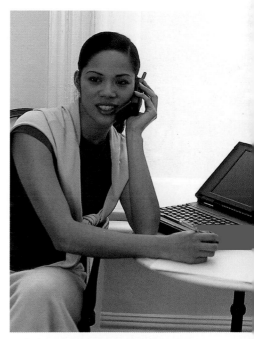

▲ *Staying confident means keeping in touch with important people in your life.*

index

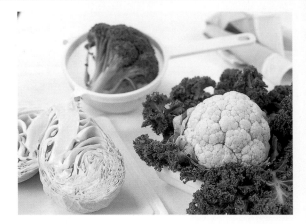

index

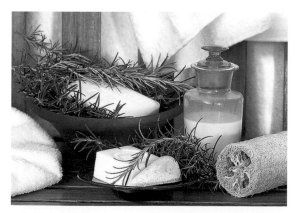

This edition is published by Lorenz Books, an imprint of Anness Publishing Ltd, Blaby Road, Wigston, Leicestershire LE18 4SE; info@anness.com

www.lorenzbooks.com; www.annesspublishing.com

If you like the images in this book and would like to investigate using them for publishing, promotions or advertising, please visit our website www.practicalpictures.com for more information.

Publisher: Joanna Lorenz
Executive Editor: Caroline Davison
Designer: Ian Sandom
Photography: Alistair Hughes, Amanda Heywood, Andrea Jones, Christine Hanscomb, Craig Robertson, Don Last, Fiona Pragoff, Janine Hosegood, John Freeman, John Heseltine, Liz McAuley, Lucy Mason, Martin Brigdale, Michelle Garrett, Sam Stowell, Sarah Cuttle, Simon Smith, Stephen Swain, Steve Moss, Steve Wooster, Sue Atkinson, Thomas Odulate, William Lingwood
Production Controller: Helen Wang

PUBLISHER'S NOTE
The reader should not regard the recommendations, ideas and techniques expressed and described in this book as substitutes for the advice of a qualified medical practitioner or other qualified professional. Any use to which the recommendations, ideas and techniques are put is at the reader's sole discretion and risk.